SECRETS OF THE BATTLE FROM A YOUNG BREAST CANCER SURVIVOR

SECRETS OF BREAST CANCER KNOWING IT EXISTS IS NOT ENOUGH.

WRITTEN BY: LAKEIA CLARK

Hi everyone,
This book is for you if you are someone fighting cancer
or very close to a cancer patient.

MEDICAL DISCLAIMER: This information and advice published or made available through www.iamlakeiaclark.com and the SECRETS OF BREAST CANCER Book are not intended to replace the services of a physician, nor does it constitute a doctor patient relationship. Information in this guide and on www.iamlakeiaclark.com is provided for informational purposes only and is not a substitute for professional medical advice. You should not use the information in this guide and on www.lakeiaclark.com for diagnosing or treating a medical or health condition. You should consult a physician in all matters relating to your health, and particularly in respect to any symptoms that may require diagnosis or medical attention. Any action on your part in response to the information provided in this ebook and on www.iamlakeiaclark.com is at the reader's discretion. Readers should consult their own physicians concerning the information in this book and on www.iamlakeiaclark.com. We make no representations or warranties with respect to any information offered or provided on or through the www.iamlakeiaclark.com web site and the SECRETS OF BREAST CANCER Book regarding treatment, action, or application of the information discussed in this book. We are not liable for any direct or indirect claim, loss or damage resulting from the use of this book, web site and/or any web site(s) linked to/from it.

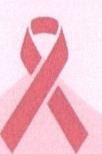

Table of Contents
Intro
My Diagnosis
My Treatment Plan
On Chemo Day What To Expect
What Happens When You Sit In The Chemo Chair
What Happens When You Get Home
Chemo Brain
Body Dryness
Hair Loss
Nail Discoloration/ Loss
Bowel & Bladder
Neutropenia: Low White Blood Cell Count
Hot Flashes & Period Loss
Neuropathy. Sensitivity to smell. Mouth Sores.
Weight Gain
Infertility
Do I Stop Working
Should I Change My Diet
Avoid Eating
Enjoy Eating
Book 3 Appointments
Surgery
Note From Me To You

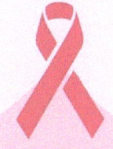

Breast Cancer has united us and now we are Breast Friends. So, I say to you
Hello Breast Friends, How are you holding up?

Let me guess, not in a million years did you think you'd be diagnosed with breast cancer huh? I definitely didn't. In fact, when I was diagnosed with breast cancer at 33 years old, I didn't even think it was possible! I remember searching online to see what to expect and being traumatized by the results. Everything scared me! I thought I was going to die. The information I saw online was either too depressing with an overload of pink ribbons and pictures of old ladies. I just couldn't relate! The best guidance I ever received was from other young breast cancer patients slightly ahead of me in treatment. They helped me to better understand my diagnosis, treatments and options way more than my own doctors (besides let's face it, we want to see if anyone else had experience and understand what we are faced with!). I want to give you that same guidance! Real and honest experiences (no fluff) with helpful tips and tricks to get you through this roller coaster ride of life's journey! After my own experience, I've learnt a lot! And lucky for you, I am willing to share my journey. I am your messenger of hope!

Please keep in mind that methods used for the treatment of breast cancer depends on the type of cancer you have and other variables specific to you. Remember, your body and spirit is unique and therefore treatments and their symptoms may vary. Please note this is NOT a medical guide to understand your prognosis. This guide is filled with real life experiences to simply give you an idea of what to expect. All so that you can make the best decisions for yourself as well as Choose Happy despite your circumstance!

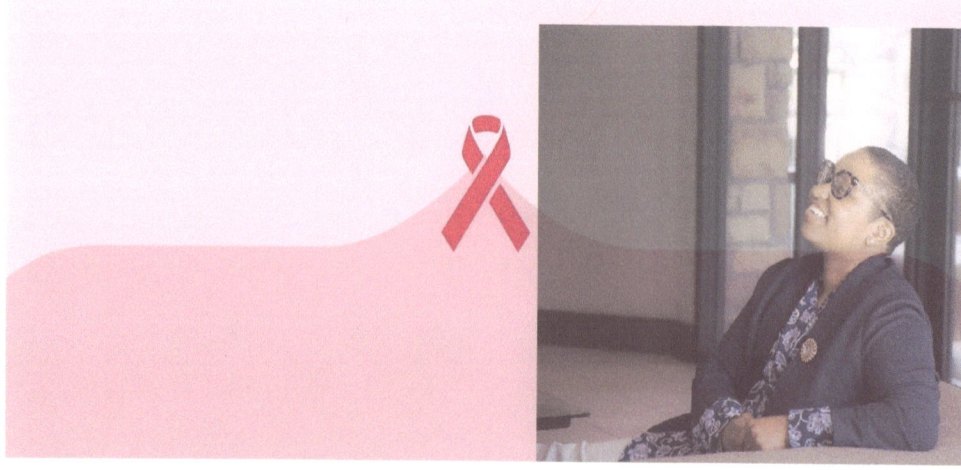

My Diagnosis

I noticed a lump in my right breast, I told my family and they insisted that I go get it checked out. Initially, I hesitated about going to the doctor as I thought maybe it was not serious. It was not until I began to have a burning sensation in my breast. It hurt so bad that it brought tears to my eyes. I called and scheduled an appointment. I went in and they did a breast exam. The doctor stated that she felt a mass. They scheduled me for a mammogram and a sonogram because of my age-33. Once the doctor reviewed the results. They insisted on a biopsy because the mass was solid. I scheduled the biopsy a week later. I went to have the biopsy done and headed home. I got in the car and just started praying, that's all I could do, leave it in Gods hands. I waited a few days and was called back in the office. That's when the doctors sat me down at a table and said you have breast cancer. I was first diagnosed August 15, 2017 with Stage 2A breast cancer. I remember being in complete shock when I was diagnosed. I have no family history of breast cancer, and I was only 33. Initially, I was suppose to have a lumpectomy and do hormone therapy. However, a week before my surgery my medical team sent me for additional testing. This is when they found out the cancer was more aggressive than they thought. So, the surgery I had scheduled was changed from an lumpectomy to the install of a mediport in order to receive chemotherapy. Things change so much that once I finished my chemo treatments, I had to have a mastectomy. I had my surgery and once the pathology report came back a week later it was determined they did not get it all. They did not clear the margins. Therefore, back in surgery I went. The second time they were able to clear all margins and there was no evidence of cancer. After healing a little, I started radiation. After about two weeks of radiation, I went back to follow up with my doctor to find out that I needed to have a year of Herceptin. I was frustrated because I was looking forward to being done active treatment. However, God has a way of sticking you in a thing and not taking you out until He is ready. What I learn is that from here on out I must look at my cancer as a chronic disease that I have to maintain. It's just like having a prescription for eyewear. You will have glasses all your life unless you have the surgery. With breast cancer, you will have to be mindful of it forever. It's just a necessary process in order to ensure our survival.

My Treatment Plan
4 cycles of Chemotherapy
Radiation
Mastectomy
Herceptin & Hormone Therapy
Reconstructive Surgery

After many treatments and surgeries later I am here, ready to share my story and spread awareness to young women like myself. If you feel something abnormal go get checked. With an early diagnosis, breast cancer is far more survivable and curable. I hope that my story and this book inspire and inform you through these difficult times. I pray everyday simply by saying Heavenly Father, I come to you as humble as I know how to give thanks for the many blessings you have bestowed upon my life. Thank You for the ups and the downs, my cloudy days, and the sunshine and rain. Most Graciously Father, you said it in your word that in order to have a Testimony you Must have a test. To have an abundance of Faith of the size of a mustered seed and believe that, I can do all things through Christ which strengthens me. (Phili 4;13). Father God when you made me the chosen vessel which was already preordained in the womb, that I will be diagnosed with stage 2 breast cancer at the of 33, I literally thought my life was over and was afraid of the possibility of dying. My mind was cloudy, my heart was broken, I felt that my health was being attack by the enemy But yet, my Faith was never shaken. I often questioned, "Why Me Lord" but God said, "Why Not You"! Don't you know that God gives his toughest battles to his strongest soldiers. In the Bible Psalm 27;1 , The Lord is my light and my salvation; whom shall I fear? The Lord is my strength of my life; whom shall I be afraid? I've trusted his process and not my diagnosis and by His Stripes, I Am Healed! As I continue to adjust to my new normal, I've grown mentally, physically, and spiritually. I know that my work isn't completed, God doesn't birth Failures. I have a purpose and I will continue to share my story.

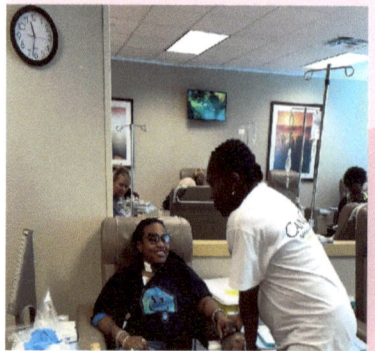
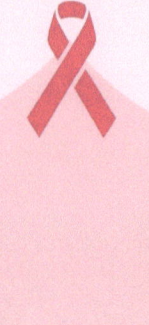
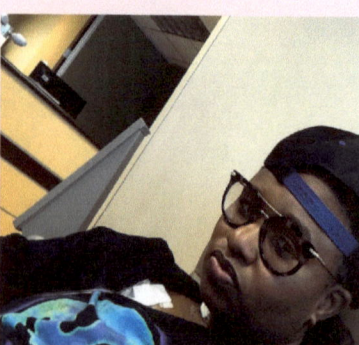

On Chemo Day What To Expect

On Chemo Day What To Expect
HOW LONG DOES IT TAKE?

I've spent up to 8 hours at the hospital! That included a blood test, oncologist appointment and long waiting hours for various reasons before treatment. On average it took a minimum of 3-4 hours. So be sure to bring some patience along with you! Remember to take your steroid pill prescribed by your doctor (the day before treatment)... you will thank me later! Here is what a typical chemo day looks like:

- You start off with a blood test to check if your white blood cell count is high enough to handle chemotherapy.
- Around thirty minutes to an hour later, once the results are in, you will either see your Oncologist for a checkup or your head nurse will verify the blood test results for you. Usually you have to see your Oncologist at least once every 3 weeks. Therefore, you see him/her before every treatment and you'll be scheduled once every 3 weeks.
- If your WBC count is high enough the nurse will give you a paper for your chemotherapy prescription and you'll have to take it to the pharmacy, where they will prepare your drugs. Sometimes, they do it for you but be sure to inquire so that you would not have to wait longer for your prescription to be prepared.
- Once everything is prepped you are ready for chemotherapy! Obviously, all hospitals function differently, but I just wanted to give you an idea of what to expect.

Our Secret:
Before you attend chemo I want you to tell yourself "This is only temporary. This is necessary. This is my new full time job! This is where I am meant to be! No where else!" Because depending on your hospital, treatments can take up to a full day. The last thing you want to do is stress yourself out by thinking of the hundreds of other things you could be doing right now. Truth is... this is exactly where you need to be! Thanks to this, all those things you dream about in the future you will have a chance to do.

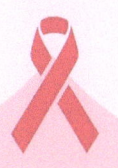
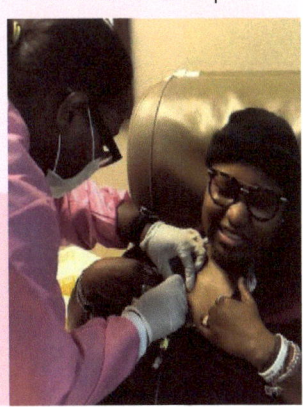

What Happens When You Sit In The Chemo Chair?

WHAT HAPPENS WHEN YOU SIT IN THE CHEMO CHAIR?

Grab some warm blankets, extra pillows and whatever else you need! As soon as you are comfy the nurse will set up your IV, through your veins, port-a-cath or picc line. Most infusion centers uses a port-a-cath. At least that is what I had placed in my chest. Depending on what chemo you're doing the nurses will come switch the bags and set the timer, then the machine does its job! At my hospital, once the bag is done, the machine will beep loudly (it can be annoying but a total relief). Prepare to be in that chair for at least 2-3 hours. Sometimes longer depending on your treatment plan. Therefore, where loose clothing and clothing that allow easy access to your port.

WHAT DOES GETTING CHEMOTHERAPY FEEL LIKE?

While you're getting chemotherapy, aside from the pinch of the needle, you don't really feel much! Every treatment was different but one thing they all had in common is that they were absolutely exhausting! Oh man... that Benadryl will knock you out! They inject it prior to chemo to avoid any allergic reactions that are common to occur. As soon as it's injected I instantly was fighting to stay awake. However, I often fell asleep! Fall asleep can help time fly by.

Other common side effects you may experience during treatment include: • Drowsiness • Weakness • Dry mouth • Dry Skin • Itchiness • Hot Flashes • Vomiting • Metallic taste in your mouth.

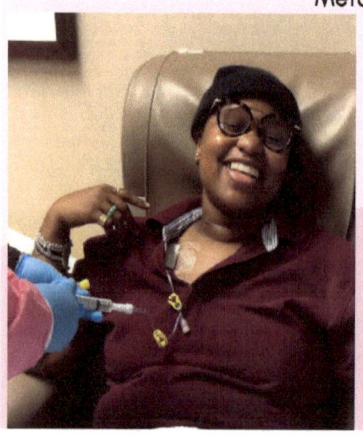
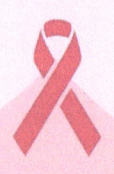
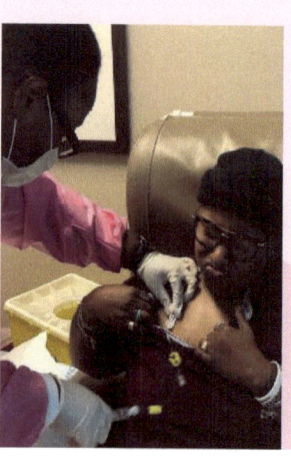

What Happens When You Get Home?

The first time I did chemotherapy as soon as I finished I felt perfectly fine! Since it was my very first treatment my mother and father came to support me. After an extremely long and overwhelming day, you may feel nauseous! Your head hurts, stomach aches and you want to puke but nothing comes out? This is how you could feel the first 24 hours after doing a round of chemotherapy. However, I must admit, I never actually vomited after chemo, I think the anti-nausea and pre medication prevents you from doing so. Therefore, as a word of advice, after chemo, please go straight home!

Asides from possible nausea for the first couple of days, you'll notice that the more chemo you do, the more likely you are to experience the following side effects.

Chemo Brain
Body Aches
Dryness
Hair Loss
Nail Discoloration/ Loss
Bowel & Bladder
Neutropenia: Low White Blood Cell Count
Hot Flashes & Period Loss
Neuropathy. Sensitivity to smell. Mouth Sores.
Weight Gain
Infertility

#1 RULE: Always discuss your side effects with your doctor. It's important that your Oncologist knows exactly how you feel, so that he/she can make any changes to your treatment or prescribe something that may help.

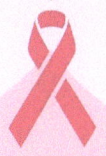

Chemo Brain

Chemo Brain. Also known as chemo fog. Basically you feel intoxicated when you just don't want to be! Everything seems foggy, fuzzy and you feel buzzed all the time. Many of my Breast Friends explained it as feeling disconnected from their body. It's not just the chemo that causes this, but also a mix of all the physical and psychological changes you're going through.

I remember when I was half way through my rounds of treatment, There I was... sitting in my chair... staring out the window completely out of it! Everyone's voice sounded like murmurs. Things I saw was blurred. It was like I was seeing straight through everything but it all appeared blurred. A few minutes passed before I snapped out of it. A couple of my Breast Friends said they became more forgetful and experienced dyslexia. Like when you walk into a room and you forget why you're there in the first place. They'd forget passwords, birthdays or even what they were saying in mid sentence. I often forget what I was saying in mid sentence.

Our Secret:
1. Drink a full bottle of water! Sometimes you may feel dizzy because you are simply dehydrated.
2. Try yoga or any type of meditation. Often hospitals offer free classes. Take advantage of them.
3. Exercise to circulate oxygen through your body and brain. This doesn't mean go to the gym and do a hardcore work out. Simply get up, walk around or climb a small flight of stairs.
4. Keep your brain active, especially when your body can't be. Write about your day in your journal, do a puzzle or cook from recipes.

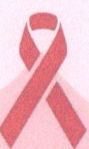

Body Aches

There will be days that you'll feel like you just got hit by a truck! Sore muscles, bones, back, ears, ankles and teeth are symptoms that we all experienced. Sore muscles might not necessarily be from the chemo itself, but it's a common side effect for other medications like Neulasta shots (to boost your WBCs when necessary) and Lupron injections (if you're trying to protect your fertility).

Our Secret:
1. Take a Tylenol to relieve the pain. But DO NOT take ibuprofen (Advil), it thins the blood! Basically do not take any anti-inflammatory drugs. Before taking a Tylenol, check your temperature. If you have a fever, it is important to call your head nurse immediately so that they can determine what is causing the fever. They may need to make adjustments to your treatments.
2. Stretch! Do simple stretching exercises or attend a yoga class.
3. Get a massage! But be sure to ask for your oncologist's permission first.
4. Hot/Cold therapy. Let's say your back is sore, Bathe your back in hot water (hot enough so it doesn't burn) for 2 minutes. And then switch to cold water for 1 minute. Repeat 3 times. This will help get the blood flowing to relieve tension and pain.

Dryness

Get ready for dry skin, eyes, mouth and vagina, which can lead to itchiness and discomfort. Unfortunately, a side effect all of us could relate to! My mouth and throat always felt dry too, like I was constantly thirsty despite having drank a full liter of water.

Our Secret:
1. Moisturize with a thick unscented cream, day and night right after you come out of the shower.
2. Chemo can make your skin sensitive to the sun, so be sure to slap on some powerful sunscreen before you go out or simply wear long sleeves and a hat.
3. Bring Visine, lip balm and hand cream with you wherever you go!
4. Drink lots of water and carry a reusable water bottle with you at all times.
5. Use water based safe lubricants and moisturizers for vaginal discomfort. Apply generously!

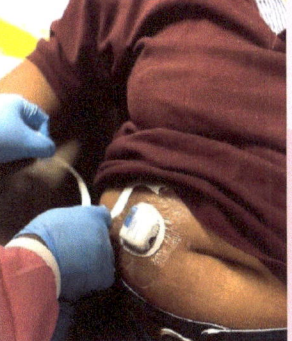
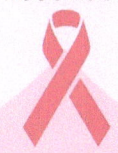

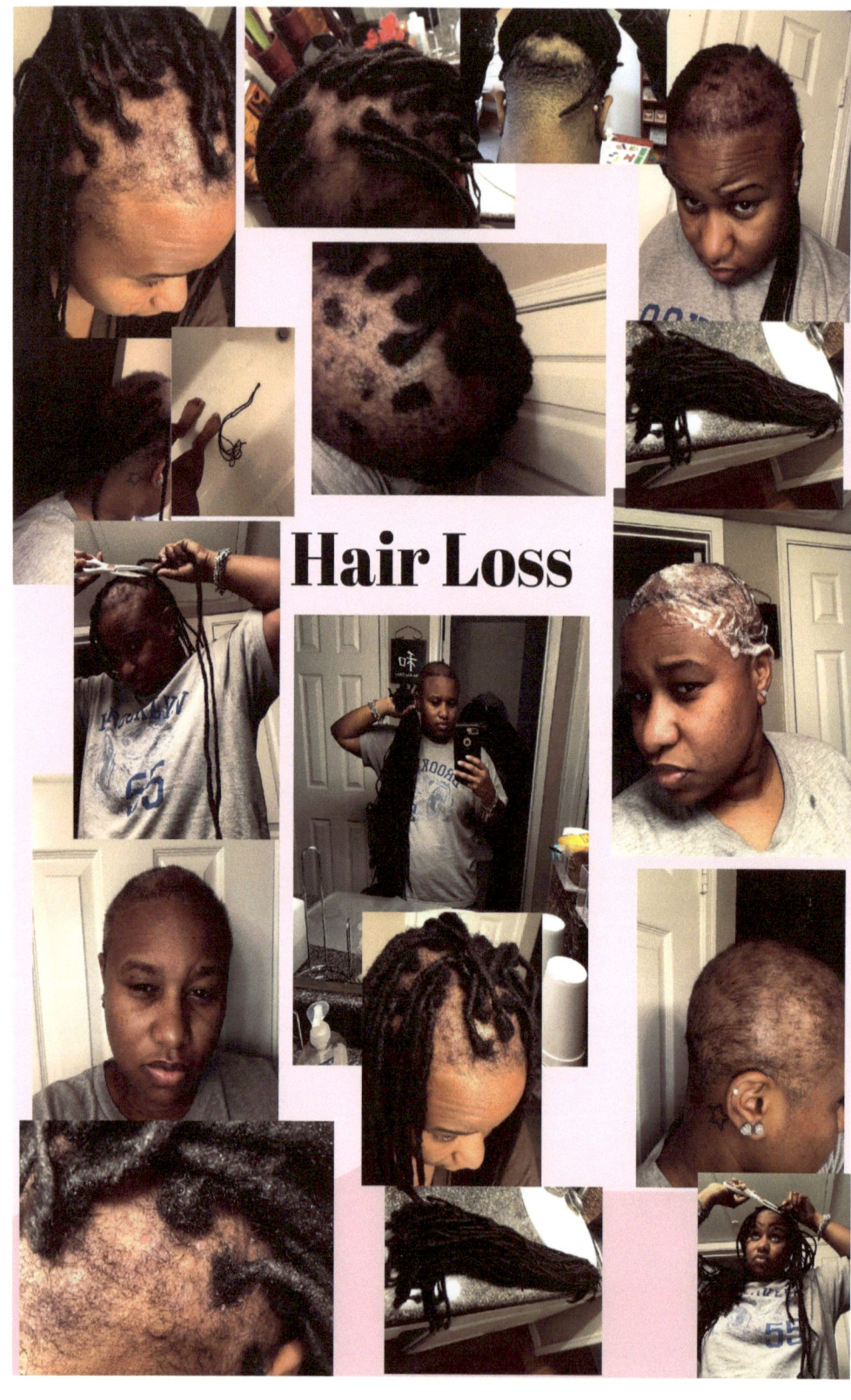

Hair Loss

When I heard that I had to have chemotherapy the thought was I do not want to lose my hair. During the process, I hated losing my hair. Exactly 15 days after the first dose I lost one dreadlock. I was standing up taking a picture and look down and their my dread was on the ground. From then on, it started to gradually fall out. Prepare for clumps of hair coming out in the shower, on your brush and in your hands as you pass your fingers through. I would just be standing and a dread would fall to the ground. This was definitely one of the most traumatic moments in my life. Even if you know it's going to happen and you try to mentally prepare yourself... seeing your hair fall out after years of growth hurts! I let the chemo do its work for weeks. My hairline kept falling out each day. I had bald patches everywhere and at some point my scalp became so irritable... I hated it. So I stopped thinking about how to preserve it, and I took action! My scalp was so irritable it kept me up all night. That same night, I decided to just let it go. I wanted my scalp to have relief and I understood that I had to get rid of the hair that remained in order to do so. All of it had to go! I grab the scissors and cut the remainder of my dreads out. I could actually pull them out if I wanted to; However, my scalp was already hurting so I just cut them out. As shocking as it was too see myself bald for the first time... I felt... relieved! I wash my hair and my scalp felt better. I got rid of remainder of my hair because it felt good. If you are going to have chemotherapy, there is no escaping the hair loss. The hair loss will begin 2-3 weeks after your first treatment. You can try to use baby shampoos, hairspray and Afro picks to gently comb your hair in order to keep it as long as possible but honestly, it's inevitable!

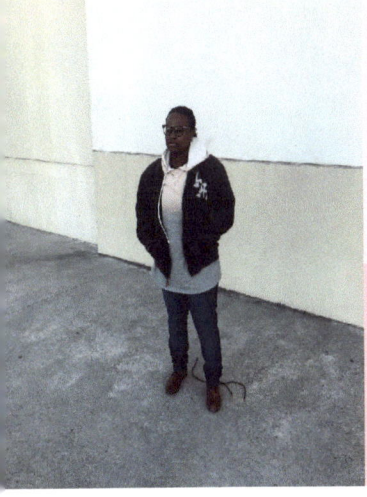
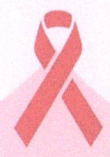

Hair Loss

Gain Control Over Your Hair Loss

1. Right before your first round, get the funkiest haircut you always wanted but never had the guts to do! My dreads used to be pass my rear end! After years of having dreads, it how I identify myself. I did not know how I would look or feel being bald. So you can imagine how hard it was to know I was going to be bald.

2. Throw a "Shaved Heads" Party! Gather your friends and family who are daring enough to join the challenge. Allow them to break the ice for you. Shave their heads first, and then ask a loved one to shave your head last! When it's all over, take lots of pictures and frame them. It's the perfect way to turn a bad memory into a good one!

3. Do a good deed: Donate it! If your hair is at least 8 inches long (tied in a ponytail from top to bottom), you should donate it! I suggest you donate it to a foundation that makes wigs for children with cancer. Knowing that your hair is going towards a good cause is bound to make you smile in the end.

WHAT'S THIS I HEAR ABOUT A COLD CAP?

Apparently, the cold cap is a device that helps prevent hair loss. I have heard several stories about the cold cap. The main one that stuck out to me was that it prevents chemotherapy from reaching cancer cells that may be in the scalp. Not only that, but you're just adding more stress and discomfort to the process. Chemo isn't fun already! So why add more to your situation? Imagine having to freeze your head just to keep your hair in "longer". Besides, with having to take chemo, you can't avoid hair loss! So my best advice is to accept the process, get through it with a smile knowing that you are Choosing Life instead of your hair. Your hair will GROW BACK when you are done treatment.

Our Secret:
1. Buy a cheap wig first to test it out. If you like it, then you can invest in a similar wig of better quality.
2. Before even buying a wig, check if your hospital has any to donate first!
3. Check if your insurance covers it! Many of my Breast Friends wigs were covered by their insurance.
4. Make the process fun! Get a hairdresser to help you out or bring your friends with you and try different styles and colors. I made a dread wig. I wore it for a while until it was to hot with the hot flashes. So, I would just put on a baseball cap. I began to accept my battle, and focus on getting better rather than worrying about covering up. But don't get me wrong! There is nothing wrong with wearing a wig. It may help you feel "normal". What's important is that you do what makes YOU feel comfortable! Do what gives you the same peace of mind that will allow you to heal. If wearing a wig brings you comfort, then by all means, rock it girl!

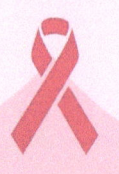
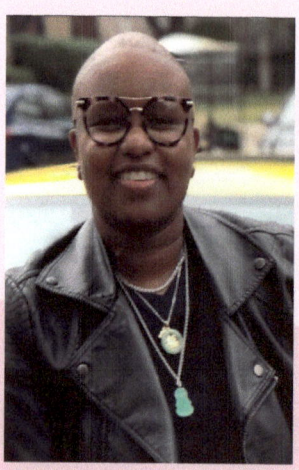

Hair Loss

Losing Your Eyebrows and Eyelashes

As soon as you lose your eyebrows and eyelashes, that's when you really start to look "sick". And when you look sick, you feel even sicker. My eyelashes and eyebrows fell out as time went by. I did not lose all of my eyebrows nor my eyelashes. It was very fine and few, but I did not lose all. Nevertheless, everywhere else I was completely hairless. On average, many individuals will lose their brows and lashes about half way through treatment. But there are a few lucky ones who will not lose them at all.

Our Secrets:

1. Wear Fake Lashes and Draw on Your Eyebrows
2. Another trick is to use eyeliner and draw a thick line at the edge of your eyelid where your lashes start. This will create an eyelash illusion.

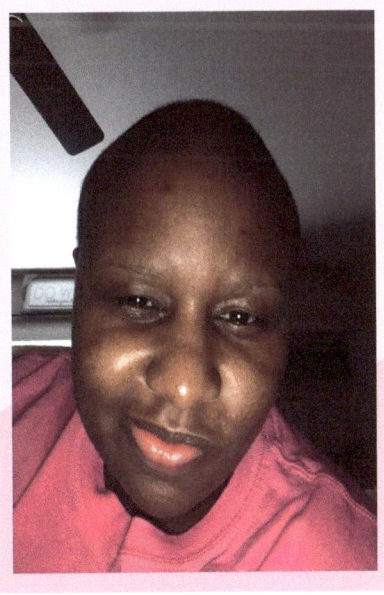
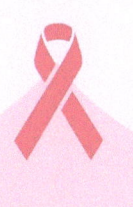
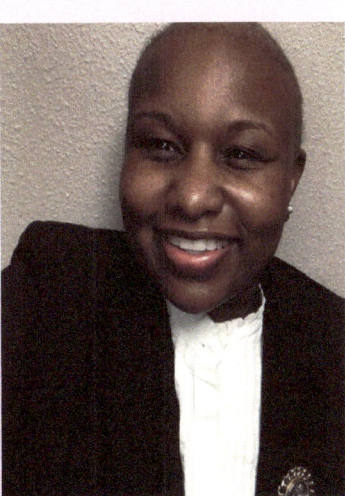

Nail Discoloration/ Loss

My nails went from yellow, to brown to completely black by the end of treatment. The sole of my feet turned black. The palm of my hands turned black. Luckily my nails did not fall off, which could have been a possibility. While this is something I experienced, my Breast Friends nails became more brittle and sore.

Our Secret:
1. Apply 100% Vitamin E Oil day and night.
You can also try sesame oil, olive oil, coconut oil or cuticle cream.
2. As much as it's tempting to wear nail polish to cover it up. DON'T! You must allow your nails to breathe and nail polish can cause more damage.
3. Cut your nails short so that they do not get caught in anything.
4. Don't worry, once you complete chemo, your dead nails will grow out and new healthy nails will grow in.

Bowel & Bladder

Good old constipation and diarrhea! I don't think you need further explanation... Certain aspects of the treatment such as medications, lack of fluids and physical activity can lead to constipation. It's so important that constipation is relieved because this can cause nausea, vomiting and stomach pain! While this may be common, it's usually not severe or long lasting. But be sure to notify your physician about diarrhea because it can lead to dehydration, lack of electrolytes and malnutrition, which in turn can delay your chemotherapy. Chemo can also irritate the lining of your bladder. So you may see blood in your urine, burning or pain when you pee or a frequent need to urinate. If this is happening, be sure to seek advice from your doctor.

Our Secret:
1. Water, water, water. I said it once; I'll say it again! Drink lots of water! You must take extra effort in hydrating yourself during these particular times.
2. Drink coconut water to get your electrolytes up and extra potassium!
3. Ask your doctor to prescribe you with laxatives or stool softeners for constipation if needed. My doctor prescribe them before treatment even start as a precaution. Before taking medicine from over the counter, to treat any of these symptoms, please ensure you consult your doctor first.

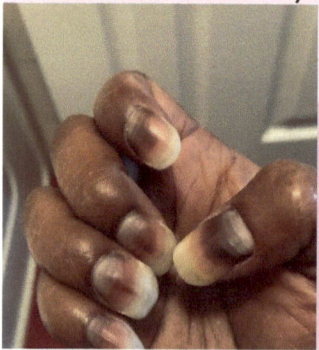
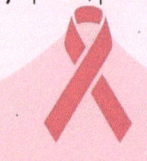
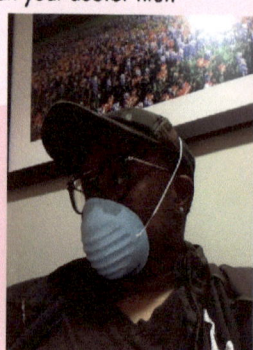

Neutropenia: Low White Blood Cell Count.

Our white blood cells are the foundation of our immune system. It's what fights infections and removes poison, waste and damaged cells from our body. When our count is low, that's when we can easily get sick. So we become prone to catching colds, flues and other diseases. What's dangerous is that it's harder for us to get better! When you're sick, your Oncologist may postpone a cycle of your chemotherapy. Something you don't want to do, because delays may make treatments less effective, and it's frustrating to have to push back your "finish line".

Our Secret:

1. If your WBC is low, stay away from public areas where you could easily catch something. For example, if you're at the movie theatre, sitting next to someone coughing and sniffling like crazy... get out of there right away! I stayed away from people and public places for at least a week and a half after treatment. I would simply do laundry, grocery shopping, etc. before my treatment every cycle.

2. Refrain from doing dangerous activities where you may get cut or bruised. When our WBC count is low it takes longer for us to heal.

3. Don't become a social butterfly either! I still went out to church and spent time with my friends on some days that I felt good. Just be careful. Wash your hands frequently and carry hand sanitizer with you. If your friends or anyone around are sick, tell them you'll see them another time!

4. Ask your doctor about Neulasta. It's an injection that will help boost your white blood cell count. My doctor gave me Neulasta after every chemo cycle.

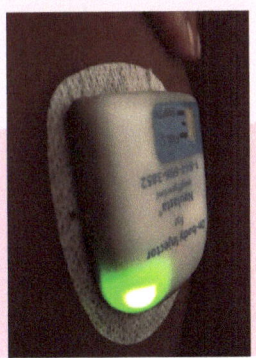
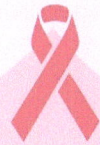

Period Loss

Whoever thought that NOT getting your period would be a bad thing? Ha! Women should be grateful for their periods I tell ya! Chemo can definitely mess with your cycle. It can even put you under menopause and stop your period temporarily. But don't worry it will come back a couple of months after you finish your last treatment.

Our Secret:
1. If you do get your period avoid tampons to prevent any infection.
2. Carry pads with you at all times, you never know when you'll randomly spot.
3. Enjoy this time off! No periods. C'mon?! That's awesome!

Since we are talking Period Loss, lets talk a little about our sex secrets:

1. Communication is key! Talk to your partner. Let them in on exactly how you feel. Don't isolate them. Our partners can easily feel powerless and vulnerable in these situations as well. It's so important to let them know it's not their fault. Once you've explained how you feel you've done your part! If they understand, they're a keeper! If they don't ... I believe everything happens for a reason and this may be your epiphany that they're probably not the one for you!
2. Try not to lose complete physical contact with your partner. If there is a decrease in sex, increase the kisses, cuddles, hugs and romance!
3. LUBE! Lube lube lube! When you're dry down there, don't force it because it can be painful. Let's try not to add pain to your already painful life ok? Slap on a safe water based lubricant and have some fun.
4. Relaxation exercises like yoga can help you loosen up!
5. If you feel unattractive, here's your special occasion to wear that wig you never wore! Dress up, wear some lingerie, put on make up, watch porn, use sex toys, and role-play! Light some candles up and play your favorite seductive slow jams. Take action and try to spice things up! Most importantly do whatever it takes for you to feel sexy. Men love women with confidence.
6. Take your time! Follow your body! Don't force yourself. Do what feels right. If it's not happening with your partner, try touching yourself or using a vibrator to keep your pleasure muscles active.
7. Hang in there! Remember this is temporary. Things do get better after treatment!

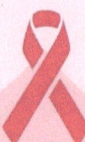

Hot Flashes

Chemo can definitely mess with your cycle. It can even put you under menopause and stop your period temporarily. But don't worry it will come back a couple of months after you finish your last treatment. Some of my Breast Friends purposely put themselves under menopause with Lupron injections to protect their fertility. Sadly, chemotherapy can make you infertile! I never thought I would get signs of menopause in my early 30s. Moreover, breast cancer. Throughout my treatment intense feelings of heat ran through my entire body at least 5 times a day! I would get hot then get cold. In traffic, in bed or during dinner! It didn't matter when or where. It happens all of a sudden. Hot flashes are one thing all of us can certainly relate to! They are mainly caused by hormonal changes and the various medication that we may take.

Our Secret:
1. Wear layers! Whenever it gets too hot, take a layer off and breath deeply.
2. Wear loose and breathable clothing such as cotton. Nothing too tight or thick. Trust me, you'll regret it.
3. Keep a cold water bottle with you at all times. Once it starts, take a sip!
4. Keep a small towel and wet ones with you. Sometimes, it's so intense your entire face starts to sweat. You're going to want to wipe your forehead and freshen up at random times.
5. Eat a popsicle or ice cream. It's refreshing!

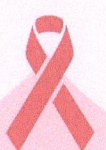

Neuropathy. Sensitivity to smell. Mouth Sores.

Neuropathy. Sensitivity to smell. Mouth Sores. Some ladies experience nerve damage in certain areas of their legs, arms, hands, feet and face. I started to feel it in my fingertips towards my final treatments. You know that feeling you get when you sit on your feet for too long and they sort of fall asleep? Yes! That numb, tingly, static feeling that we all hate! That's what it feels like! For me, it would come and go.

But here's the One & Only Secret: If you start experiencing neuropathy it is extremely important that you mention this to your nurse or oncologist RIGHT AWAY so that they can either delay or decrease the treatment, as this can become permanent. Don't wait until it gets worse. I repeat, if you experience any signs of neuropathy you must seek advice from your doctor immediately.

Sensitivity to smell. Mouth Sores.

It's funny how a lot of the symptoms that pregnant women experience, are similar to us breast cancer patients. Like forgetfulness and the sensitivity to smell. You will realize perfumes will smell stronger than usual and scents that you used to love may make you feel nauseous.

Our Secret:

Carry a small bottle of lavender oil with you. Whenever you smell something that makes you feel nauseous, take a whiff! Other than that, you should avoid scented products as much as possible.

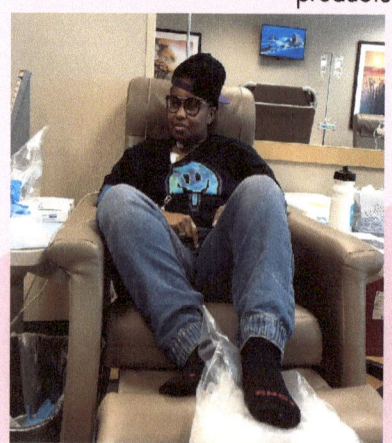
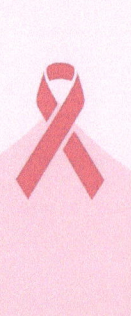
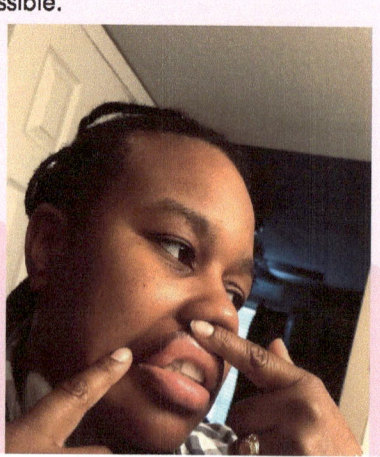

Mouth Sores.

Along with the dryness, you may get mouth ulcers or sensitive gums. This is a crucial time for you to take extra care of your dental hygiene.

Our Secret:

1. Use an extra soft bristle toothbrush and Sensodyne toothpaste. I actually used childrens tooth paste and gargle with warm salt water.
2. Never use mouthwash, use warm water mixed with baking soda or gargle with Biotene. Be sure to rinse day and night.
3. Visit your dentist before and after chemo but not during as it may cause infections. You need a dental clearance before you start treatment.

Bad Appetite. Insomnia.

Chemo can change your taste buds. Sometimes the food that you used to love will no longer taste the same. What used to be sweet, salty and spicy may seem bitter and dull. It might be harder to sleep at night for various reasons. I found myself wide-awake at night because I'd sleep too much during the day. My Breast Friends felt anxious, stressed or depressed. We have to admit; the times we tend to analyze everything we're going through, is when we're lying in bed, trying to fall asleep.

Our secrets:

1. Try to add some extra spice to your food.
2. Use plastic utensils instead of metal ones to get rid of that nasty, bitter and metallic taste that you may already have in your mouth.
3. Eat smaller portions more frequently instead of big meals.

Our secrets for Insomnia:

1. Drink chamomile tea before bed.
2. Take Melatonin. (ask your doctor first)
3. Meditate.
4. Exercise more in the day so you are more tired at night.
5. Play soothing music.

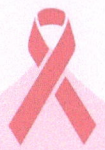

Weight Gain

Now, a lot of people think of chemotherapy and think of weight loss! We see it on television and advertisements all the time, the skinny frail patient withering away. I thought maybe that would be me. However, my doctor ensure me that I would not have that problem. I wondered why was she so confident about me not having weight loss. Well, it was because she had me taking steroids a day before my treatment and several days afters. Hello, weight gain!

Our Secrets:

1. Keep active! I still tried doing low intensity workouts at home. But be sure to follow your body. If you're weak, then a mid day walk goes a long way.
2. Watch what you eat! You already have poison in your body! Don't add junk to it. Avoid refined sugars and fast food. Once I was diagnosed, my doctor suggested that I change to a plant base diet in order to navigate the medical space with least amount of side effects, best results, and to help control my weight. Especially since fat produces estrogen, and my cancer was estrogen positive.
3. Help your body out! Eat a healthy diet. Increase your greens and proteins! I became a Vegan.
4. Accept your body now, work with it and when you're done, we'll talk about getting you back into shape later.

Weight Loss

It is not unlikely to have weight loss. However, you should consult with your doctor because weight loss can be dangerous. In some cases, weight loss may be required by your medical team, but it should not stem from your medication. Again, fat can cause more estrogen to be produce which can cause cancer. So, consult with the doctor!

Our Secrets:

1. Eat more nuts and pasteurized cheese! Not junk! Better yet Vegan Cheese!
2. If you're losing weight because you don't have an appetite, try eating smaller portions more frequently.
3. Drink Ensure.
4. If you don't have an appetite. Make yourself a smoothie! Blend some spinach, kale, blueberries, strawberries, non-dairy yogurt and almond milk. Yum!

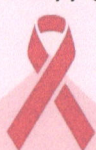

Infertility

EGG PRESERVATION LUPRON INJECTIONS

The procedure consists of retrieving your eggs, maturing them in the lab and freezing them for future use. There's also another way, such as taking an injection a few weeks before so that your eggs mature inside of you instead. It's a more complex surgery but it increases the chances of fertilization. My cancer was aggressive and I needed to start chemo right away, so there was no time to delay. I could not have this procedure because it was not in my best interest at that point. Considering the time it takes to prepare for the preservation and the aggressiveness of my cancer I made the decision to not go through with it at all, prioritizing their lives before anything. Some of my Breast Friends agreed to take Lupron injections to put them in medical menopause. It was one injection for every month of chemotherapy. Their theory suggests that if your body is under menopause you won't have any eggs, therefore there is less of a chance for chemo to harm them! Get ready for extreme hot flashes! Did you know that chemo can affect your fertility? Are you going to preserve your eggs? I would suggest that you ask your Oncologist about it right before you start chemotherapy. So, they can schedule you an appointment at the Reproductive Center. You do not want to take a risk if being a mother someday is one of your biggest dreams. Keep in mind that egg preservation can cost thousands of dollars. Because of how expensive it is many of my Breast Friends decided that it just wasn't worth it, especially since results aren't even guaranteed. The thought of not having children of my own bothers me occasionally. However, every women no matter what still have the potential of being a mother. There are other ways to be a mother if you decide not to have egg preservation and can not have any children in the future.

Our Secrets:

1. Deciding on whether or not you should preserve your eggs and take Lupron injections can be an extremely tough decision! Ask yourself this: "How important is it for you to have babies of your own in the future?" Now visualize your doctor some day telling you "Sorry, you are infertile." How does that make you feel? You can decide to do everything you can to ensure you do not become infertile. The rest will be in God's hands. If God want to use you as a vessel to bring a child into the world He will regardless of your treatment plans.

2. Knowledge is power! Do your research and ask lots of questions to know your best option. I think the decision is a personal one. One that you and your partner (should you be in a relationship) should openly discuss together.

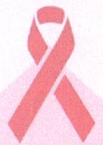

Do I Stop Working

Having to stop work was a big deal for me. Initially, I wanted to work to continue to provide for myself. However, my body would not allow with the treatment I was receiving. My employer was very supportive and lenient giving me the choice to take a leave of absence. I was only part-time anyway. The other time was me focusing on my own business. Chemotherapy treatments are unpredictable and you just never know how you're going to feel. Also, your immune system is bound to be weak, so if your work environment isn't disinfected at all times you may be at risk of getting sick! Working was a no brainer for me. As a child photographer, I was definitely going to be around germs. I personally made the choice to stop working right before I started treatment so that I could focus 100% on healing. I understand how money can be an issue for many. Hell, it was for me. Nevertheless, I believed God would make a way and He continues to provide for me.

Some of my Breast Friends continued to work during their entire treatment. Some decided to go in 1-2 days when they felt good enough, claiming it helped them feel "normal". Others had the ability to work from home! But like me, the majority decided to stop working completely and focus on themselves. So there are options! You need to choose what's right for you and don't feel bad about your choice!

Our Secrets:

1. Follow your body! Health comes first. If you have the chance to stop working and focus on healing, I highly suggest you do just that!

2. Empower yourself! Contact your insurance; you'll be surprised by what they can offer.

3. Be honest with your employer. Let them in on exactly how you feel. As much as it sucks to admit that you are sick and have to inquire about "disability" when you never imagined you'd be "disabled" (I hated even using that word), tell them everything and don't be scared to ask questions.

4. If you stop working, find a hobby! Keep your mind active. So you know that thing you've always wanted to do but never had the time to do it? NOW'S THE TIME!!!†

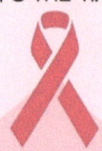

Shoud I Change My Diet

There are numerous theories and remedies for the best breast cancer prevention diets. My doctors specifically told me in order to have least amount of side effects and to navigate the medical space with not many issues, I should transition to a plant base diet. Once the doctor told me this, I stop eating meat and by product of animals immediately. So, What's my best advice for you? Well, first and foremost, it's important that you do what YOU want to do and what YOU believe works! In my case, I just place my faith in God and the doctor. What I suggest is that you eat a healthy and balanced diet. Remember, right now your body is going through a beating. You literally have poison flowing through your veins. So, I recommend you DON'T add any more crap to it. You want to help your body repair itself, but not too much so that it inhibits the chemotherapy from doing it's job. Sounds ironic huh? Trust me! I struggled with the idea!

Not only that, but your immune system is low, so there are certain foods that are usually good for you but that you need to avoid during chemotherapy treatment due to your weakened immune system.

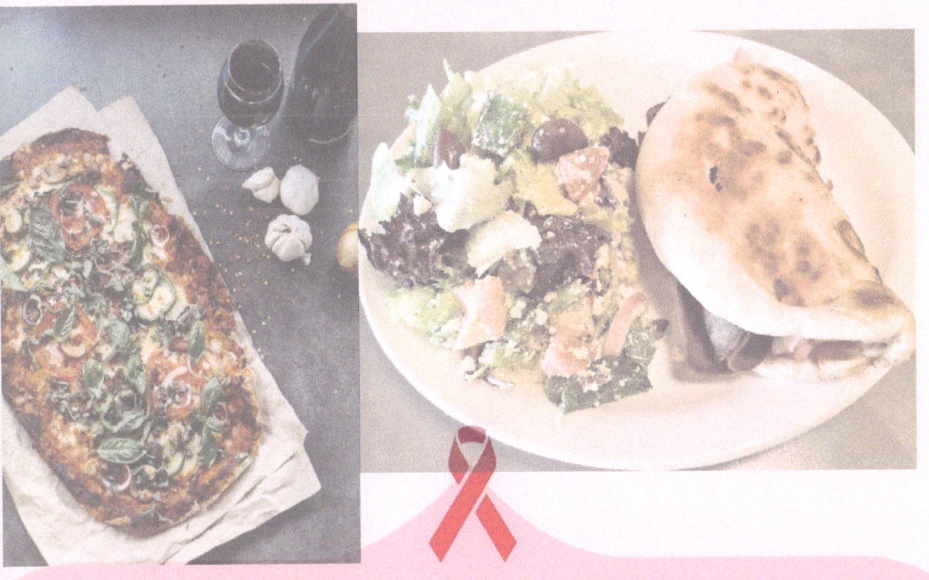

Avoid Eating

Avoid: Sushi: sorry, your body can't handle raw food right now.
- Unpasteurized cheese: contains high levels of bacteria.
- Yogurt with pro-biotics: pro-biotics contain bacteria.
- Alcohol: you have enough poison in your system. Don't add more.
- Grapefruit: Grapefruit juice can interfere with the works of chemo.
- Green Tea: Same thing for green tea. It's that powerful of a detox that it can interfere with the chemo. In other words, once you're done chemo, drink up that green tea and eat your grapefruit!
- Soy: Especially if you are hormone positive, avoid soy as it contains high concentrations of isoflavones that has estrogen-like effects.
- Sugar: the most dangerous ingredient in the world. The number one cause to several diseases. Need I say more?
- Salad Bars, buffets, and street food: Higher risk of improperly stored or refrigerated food and poor hygiene by the people handling and cooking the food. If you get food poisoning, it won't be easy to recover.

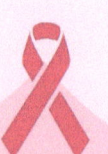

Enjoy Eating

Dark leafy greens: Be sure to wash them thoroughly.
- Less meat: When you eat meat, eat organic meat! Grass fed. No hormones.
- Fruits & Veggies: your body needs more vitamins and nutrients more than ever.
- Small portions: Get used to eating a little bit several times a day, instead of 3 big portions. It will help prevent nausea, and it's easier for your weak stomach to digest smaller portions.
- Drink fresh juices and smoothies: When you're sick, it's exhausting to have to chew on kale and spinach. But this shouldn't be an excuse to not get your daily dose of nutrients. Invest in a juicer or blender. Make fresh juices or smoothies for that much needed boost of energy.
- Drink Coconut Water

Seriously though, you're going through enough during chemotherapy that it's so important to indulge. Here's my rule. Eat healthy 80% of the time. Save 20% to indulge in your favorite cheat meals and desserts. You deserve it!

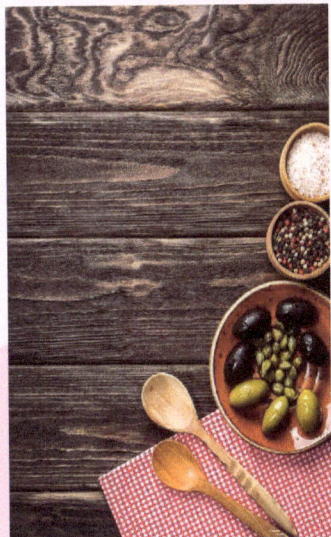
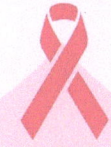

Book 3 Appoinments

3 APPOINTMENTS TO BOOK BEFORE STARTING CHEMO:

1. Dentist
We all know by now that chemo kills the good cells along with the bad. This includes the cells in your mouth. This can cause gum, teeth and gland problems. If you go to the dentist before chemotherapy begins you can help prevent serious mouth problems. Side effects often happen only if your mouth isn't healthy to begin with. It's better to get rid of any problems before, because if you get an infection you may not be able to keep up with your treatment. Your doctor may need to cut back on the chemo or even stop it.

2. Obstetrician
If having babies in the future is important to you. Book an appointment with an Obstetrician or ask your Oncologist for a referral to discuss egg preservation. Once you start chemo, it will be too late.

3. Nutritionist
It's always good to talk to a professional to get recommendations for a healthy diet based on YOUR personal needs. Perhaps you're gaining weight, losing weight, feeling dehydrated or weak. A nutritionist can help set up a healthy meal plan specific for you!

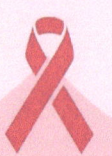

Surgery

Again everyone goes through different treatment plans. Initially I was only suppose to have a lumpectomy, but things change and I had to have a mastectomy. Under certain circumstances, people with breast cancer have the opportunity to choose between total removal of a breast (mastectomy) and breast-conserving surgery (lumpectomy) followed by radiation.

Lumpectomy followed by radiation is likely to be equally as effective as mastectomy for people with only one site of cancer in the breast and a tumor under 4 centimeters. Clear margins are also a requirement (no cancer cells in the tissue surrounding the tumor). For some women, removing the entire breast provides greater peace of mind ("just get the whole thing out of there!") as well as best course of treatment due to size and other determining factors. . Radiation therapy may still be needed, depending on the results of the pathology following the mastectomy. I had to have radiation as well. I did 33 sessions after the healing of my mastectomy.

All women heal differently. My advice will be consult with your doctor and follow their instructions both pre surgery and post surgery.

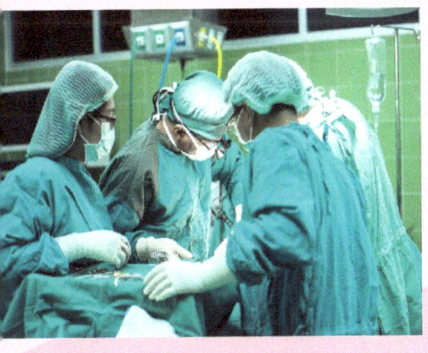
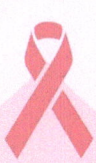
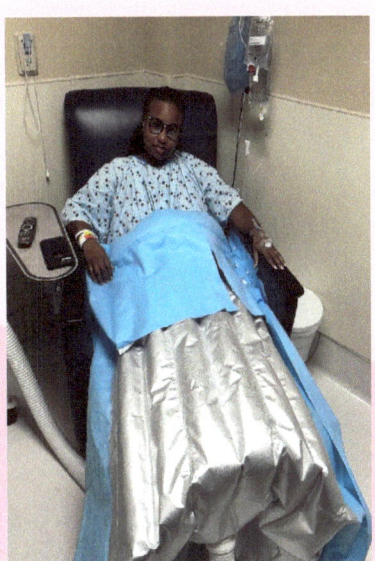

A NOTE FROM ME TO YOU

To All My Readers,

Find your Why? Find you motivation to fight. My Why was simple. I wanted to live. I wanted to be here. I felt lit was not over for me. I still have much to accomplish. Besides, I believed that God would heal my body if I did my part which was fight and do what my doctors required of me. He would stand by his word that He would protect me.

My message to other cancer patients is fight. To the family and friends of the cancer patients fight and continue to be support. I would say to the cancer patient fight to live for you and your love ones. It's not over. You still have life. Change the lens in which you view your cancer. Look at your diagnosis not as an obstacle but an opportunity. You have the ability to respond to your situation either negatively or positively. I had a choice on how I responded. I Choose Happy despite of.. Hell, this entire process was not what I wanted to endure. Yet, it was necessary in order to live after being diagnosed with breast cancer. Some things we go through in life will not feel good but will be essential to our survival. So, keep pushing because you need you. I pray that this book has been resourceful and helpful to you. Thank you for the support and purchase of this book. Remember "Life is much better when you Choose Happy. Despite your uncontrollable circumstances you have the choice to Choose Happy and to Choose Life."~ Lakeia Clark

Best Regards

Lakeia Clark

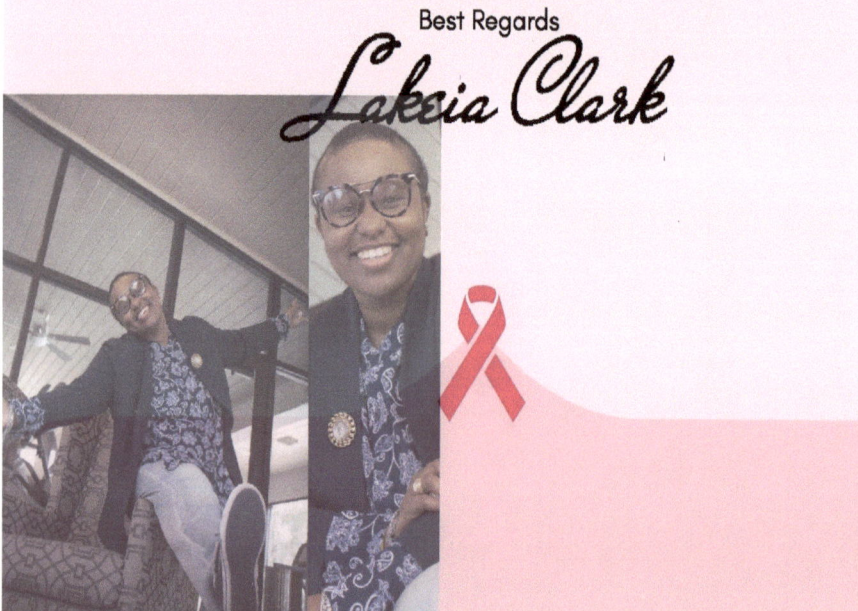

www.ingramcontent.com/pod-product-compliance
Lightning Source LLC
Chambersburg PA
CBHW040303220526
45473CB00002B/565